LEAN MUSCLE RECIPES

25 Meals For People Who Are Serious About Building Muscle

Clark Moraign

Copyright © 2015 All Right Reserved.

No part of this publication may be reproduced, distributed, or transmitted in any form or by any means, including photocopying, recording, or other electronic or mechanical methods, or by any information storage and retrieval system without the prior written permission of the publisher, except in the case of very brief quotations embodied in critical reviews and certain other noncommercial uses permitted by copyright law.

Table of Contents

Introduction
1. Lean Beefy Body Spinach Meatball and Wheat Pasta
2. Crazy Stuffed Chicken Breast with Brown Rice
3. Bicep Blasting Baked Salmon with Grilled Asparagus
4. Caramel Protein Bar Banana Split and Protein Ice Cream
5. Protein Powder, Blueberry, Banana and Oatmeal Pancakes
6. Lean and Mean Smoothie
7. Amino Acid and Protein Popsicles
8. Pre Pump Salad
9. Cardio Curry Shrimp on Rice
10. Olympic Chicken
11. Spinach, Cottage Cheese and Rice
12. Tuna Twist Salad
13. Clark's Sloppy Burger
14. Muscle Building Broccoli Salad
15. Lean Machine Trout Almandine
16. Buff Guy Chicken in White Wine Sauce
17. Crazy Blueberry and Cottage Cheese
18. Forearm Blasting Spinach Noodle Lasagna
19. Eggs over Veggies
20. Dude's Spinach Helper
21. Chili Challenge
22. Tricep Blasting Tuna Salad and Dill
23. Lean Muscle Building Grilled Steak and Cheese
24. Insane Truffles
25. Ripped Body Salmon Steaks and Quinoa
Conclusion

Introduction

First, I want to thank you for purchasing Lean Muscle Building Recipes. If you are active or workout like I do, you know how important it is to get high quality natural protein in your diet not only to maintain your muscle but to build more muscle. Supplements are fine but I tend to believe that our bodies know how to deal with natural proteins better then man made, Don't get me wrong, I do like my whey protein shakes with some amino acid powder added in the mix, along with some fruits, which is why I added some recipes in this book that use powdered proteins and amino acids and a few others. Do not feel like you need to use the exact same name brand products that are in here, you can use what you have on hand or what every high quality protein and amino acid powder you can find. I did however leave links in the back of the book that you may want to use. I searched for the best source of proteins and amino acids I could find on Amazon. Again I hope you enjoy this book and share these awesome recipes with your family members and friends

Enjoy!

1. Lean Beefy Body Spinach Meatball and Wheat Pasta

Ingredients

FOR MEATBALLS:

6 oz lean ground beef

1/2 cup shredded raw spinach

1/4 cup diced red onion

1 tbsp minced garlic

1/2 tbsp cumin

Sea salt and pepper, to taste

FOR PASTA:

2 oz wheat spinach pasta

1/8 cup marinara

1 1/2 cup raw spinach

5 cherry tomatoes

1 tbsp low fat parmesan cheese

Directions

1. Set oven to 405 degrees F.

2. Saute the red onions in a skillet using spray olive or coconut oil.

3. Mix together ground beef, chopped raw spinach, red onion, garlic, and spices. Mix thoroughly using your hands until the spinach is completely mixed into the meat.

4. Form two or three meatballs of roughly the same size using your hands. For accuracy, you can use a food scale to weigh and measure each portion.

5. Place meatballs on a baking sheet and bake in the oven for 10-12 minutes.

6. Cook pasta and stir in tomatoes, spinach, and cheese as desired.

7. Mix in cooked meatballs and enjoy!

NUTRITION FACTS

Amount per serving

Calories 468

Total Fat 6g

Total Carbs 50g

Protein 51g

2. Crazy Stuffed Chicken Breast with Brown Rice

Ingredients

6 oz. chicken breast

1/2 cup raw spinach

1 Roma tomato

2 tbsp feta cheese

1/2 cup brown rice

Directions

1. Set oven to 375 degrees F.

2. Slice the chicken breast down the middle; be careful not to slice all the way through the chicken breast.

3. Season the chicken breast with your choice of seasonings.

4. Open the chicken breast and, on one side, layer spinach, tomato slices, and feta cheese.

5. Fold the chicken breast and use toothpicks to hold the chicken breast closed.

6. Bake for 18-20 minutes or until the chicken breast is completely cooked.

7. Cook brown rice and add garlic and diced onion for extra flavor.

8. Plate chicken and brown rice.

NUTRITION FACTS

Amount per serving

Calories 363

Total Fat 6g

Total Carbs 32g

Protein 43g

3. Bicep Blasting Baked Salmon with Grilled Asparagus

Ingredients

5 oz wild salmon (Raw)

FOR MARINADE:

1 tbsp dijon mustard

1/2 tbsp olive oil

1 tsp minced garlic

Juice from half of a lemon

1 1/2 cup grilled asparagus

1/2 tbsp minced garlic

Directions

1. Set oven to 405 degrees F.

2. In a bowl, mix mustard, olive oil, garlic, and lemon juice.

3. Pour the marinade over the salmon to completely cover it. For better flavor, place the marinating salmon in the fridge for at least one hour.

4. Place the salmon on a baking sheet and top with slices of lemon (if desired). Bake for 10-12 Minutes.

5. Cut the bottom stems off the asparagus spears.

6. Set a nonstick skillet on medium high heat and lightly spray with coconut or olive oil.

7. Place the asparagus and garlic in the skillet and sear for about 5 minutes, rolling the asparagus so that all sides are seared.

8. Place asparagus with salmon on a plate and eat up!

NUTRITION FACTS

Amount per serving

Calories 282

Total Fat 16g

Total Carbs 7g

Protein 32g

4. Caramel Protein Bar Banana Split With Protein Ice Cream

Ingredients

FOR ICE CREAM:

7 oz Greek yogurt

1/2 scoop any protein powder vanilla ice cream (high protein)

1 tbsp vanilla extract

1/2 Caramel Protein Bar (any brand, high protein bar)

1 medium-large sized banana

Optional: 3 chopped/diced strawberries

Directions

1. Place Caramel Protein Bar in the freezer or refrigerator.

2. In a bowl, mix Greek yogurt, protein ice cream powder, and vanilla extract. Whip until completely smooth.

3. Place the bowl in the refrigerator for 1.5-2 hours or until desired firmness is reached.

4. Slice a banana in half vertically and place in a bowl.

5. Place Protein bar in blender and pulse until it breaks into chunks.

6. Remove the ice cream from the freezer. Using an ice cream scoop, dig out the ice cream and place on top of the cut banana.

NUTRITION FACTS

Amount per serving

Calories 493

Total Fat 12g

Total Carbs 49g

Protein 47g

5. Protein Powder, Blueberry, Banana and Oatmeal Pancakes

Ingredients

1 scoop lean high protein powder (unflavored)

1/2 cup egg whites (or 3 egg whites)

1/2 cup oatmeal (uncooked)

1/2 medium banana

1/2 cup blueberries

2 tsp baking powder

Directions

1. Place raw, uncooked oatmeal in a blender or food processor and blend until it becomes fine flour.

2. Add eggs, banana, protein powder, and baking powder and pulse blend until smooth.

3. Toss blueberries into the batter and mix using a spatula or spoon.

4. Place a skillet on medium-high heat and measure out about 1/8 cup or 2 tbsp of batter per pancake.

5. Cover the pancakes while they cook to help the inside cook faster. Cook them for about 45 seconds to 1 minute on the first side, and then about 30-45 sec on the other side.

NUTRITION FACTS

Amount per serving
Calories 544
Total Fat 11g
Total Carbs 64g
Protein 47g

6. Lean and Mean Smoothie

Ingredients

1 scoop any lean muscle protein powder (unflavored)

1 cup chopped kale

1/2 small avocado

1/3 banana

1/4 cup pineapple

3 strawberries (raw or freshly frozen)

Small bundle of wheat grass (about 1/4 oz)

1/4 cup water

Ice for desired thickness

OPTIONAL INGREDIENTS:

1/4 cup uncooked oatmeal for added heartiness

1/2 celery stalk

Directions

1. Add ingredients to a blender and mix until smooth.

2. Freeze the fruit to chill the smoothie or add ice

NUTRITION FACTS
Amount per serving
Calories 401
Total Fat 14g
Total Carbs 45g
Protein 26g

7. Amino IV and Protein Popsicles

Ingredients

1 Scoop Amino IV Cherry limeade
Or use any flavored amino acid powder you like.

1.5 scoop any lean muscle protein powder (unflavored)

1.5 cup blueberries or blackberries (or mixture of two)

1 cup chopped strawberries

1/3 cup raspberries

1/2 cup Greek yogurt

1 medium banana

6 three-ounce Dixie cups

6 popsicle sticks

Directions

1. Add 1 scoop of Amino IV to a blender.

2 Add strawberries and raspberries to the powdered and blend until smooth.

3 Pour contents into a cup or bowl and set aside.

4. Add blueberries (or blackberries) to the blender and blend until

5. Pour contents into a cup or bowl and set in the refrigerator.

6. Add banana, Greek yogurt, and Lean Muscle Protein Powder to the blender and blend until smooth.

7. Pour the contents into a cup or bowl and set aside in the refrigerator.

8. Pour Amino IV Chery Limeade flavored (or any flavored Amino acids you desire) and strawberry mixture evenly into the six Dixie cups. Place cups in the freezer for about one hour.

9. Remove the Dixie cups from the freezer and place popsicle sticks vertically into the cups.

10. Add the banana protein mixture evenly between the cups and then top with blueberry mixture. Each cup should have three layers.

11. Place in the freezer for at least four hours.

NUTRITION FACTS
Serving Size (1popsicle)
Amount per serving
Calories 114
Total Fat 1g
Total Carbs 20g
Protein 9g

8. Pre Workout Salad

Ingredients

1 cup lettuce, torn into bite-sized pieces
1/3 cup spinach, torn into bite-sized pieces
1/3 cucumber, peeled and sliced
1/3 tomato, sliced
3/4 cup sprouts
1/3 cup shredded carrots
1/3 cup sliced mushrooms
1/3 avocado, cubed
1 tbsp raw sunflower seeds
1 tbsp olive oil
2 tsp lemon juice
Dash each of thyme, parsley, basil

Directions

1. In a medium-sized salad bowl, combine lettuce, spinach, cucumber, tomato, sprouts, carrots, mushrooms, avocado, and sunflower seeds.

2. In a screw-top jar, mix olive oil with lemon juice and herbs. Shake vigorously, and pour over salad.

NUTRITION FACT

Recipe yields 2 servings
Amount per serving
Calories 167

Total Fat 9 g
Total Carb 9 g
Protein 5 g
Sodium 22 mg

9. Cardio Curry Shrimp on Rice

Ingredients

2 cups cooked rice
Dash oregano
Dash salt
1 pound large shrimp, cooked and peeled
Dash curry powder
Dash cayenne pepper
1 tomato, sliced

Directions

1. Sprinkle rice with oregano and dash of salt.

2. Sprinkle shrimp with curry powder and cayenne pepper.

3. Surround shrimp with rice and sliced tomatoes and serve.

NUTRITION FACTS

Recipe yields 4 servings
Amount per serving
Calories 223
Total Fat 1.2 g
Total Carb 28 g
Protein 23 g

10. Olympic Chicken

Ingredients

4 8-ounce chicken breasts, skinned
1/2 cup unbleached flour
1 tblsp olive oil
1/4 tsp pepper
1 4-ounce can sliced pineapple (in its own juices)
1/2 cup water
3/4 cup cider vinegar
1/4 tsp ground ginger
1 green pepper, cut into 1/4 inch rings

Directions

1. Wash and dry chicken and coat with flour.

2. in a nonstick skillet, heat oil and brown chicken.

3. Place chicken in shallow roasting pan.

4. Sprinkle with pepper.

5. Make sauce of pineapple juice, water, vinegar, and ginger.

6. Pour over chicken and bake, uncovered, in a 350 degree oven for 30 minutes.

7. Add pineapple slices and green pepper rings. Cook for 15 minutes and serve.

NUTRITION FACTS

Recipe yields 4 servings
Amount per serving
Calories 291
Total Fat 39 g
Total Carb 14 g
Protein 39 g

11. Spinach, Cottage Cheese and Rice

Ingredients

1/3 cup rice, cooked
3 tbsp low-fat cottage cheese
1 egg white, beaten until fluffy
2 tsp chopped fresh parsley
2 tsp chopped fresh dill
Dash of pepper
2 cups fresh spinach, chopped
3 tsp whole-wheat bread crumbs

Directions

1. Preheat oven to 350 degrees.

2. In a mixing bowl, combine rice and cottage cheese in a small bowl, mix together egg white, parsley, dill, and pepper.

3. Add spinach and egg white mixture to rice mixture. Mix well. Pour into casserole dish, and sprinkle bread crumbs on top.

4. Bake for 40 minutes.

NUTRITION FACTS

Recipe yields 2 servings
Amount per serving
Calories 157
Total Fat 1g

Total Carb 29g
Protein 7g
Sodium 113mg

12. Tuna Twist Salad

Ingredients

1 pear, chopped
1 slice pineapple, chopped
1 7-ounce can water-packed tuna, flaked and drained
1/2 cup low-fat yogurt
1/2 tsp curry powder
1/2 tsp vanilla
1/4 cup raisins
1 apple, chopped
Lettuce leaves

Directions

1. Mix all ingredients except lettuce, tossing until well combined.

2. Line a large plate with lettuce leaves.

3. Arrange mixture on lettuce leaves and serve chilled.

NUTRITION FACTS

Recipe yields 2 servings
Amount per serving
Calories 345
Total Fat 2.8 g
Total Carb 51 g
Protein 33 g

13. Clark's Sloppy Burger

Ingredients

1 pound ground sirloin tip
1 16-ounce can Ragu cooking sauce
1/4 tsp oregano
1/4 tsp basil
1/4 tsp thyme
Dash hot red pepper
Dash black pepper
1/8 tsp chili powder
4 whole wheat pita rounds

Directions

1. Brown meat in a skillet and drain all fat.

2. Pour Ragu cooking sauce onto meat and simmer for 5 minutes with oregano, basil, thyme, hot pepper, black pepper, and chili powder.

3. Spoon into whole wheat pita rounds and serve.

NUTRITION FACTS

Recipe yields 4 servings
Amount per serving
Calories 263
Total Fat 11.8 g
Total Carb 21 g
Protein 28.4 g

14. Muscle Building Broccoli Salad

Ingredients

1/2 pound cooked steak, cut in strips
1 cup broccoli, cooked and chopped
1 cup green beans, cooked and cut
1 stalk celery, sliced
1/2 cup mushrooms, sliced
1 green onion, sliced
1/2 tbsp red wine vinegar
1/2 tbsp lemon juice
1/4 cup nonfat yogurt
1/2 tsp mustard
1/4 tsp ground pepper
1/2 head of lettuce
1/2 tomato, sliced
Fresh parsley

Directions

1. In large salad bowl, combine steak, broccoli, green beans, celery, mushrooms, and onion.

2. In a screw-top jar, combine the vinegar, lemon juice, yogurt, mustard, and pepper, and shake until thoroughly mixed for the salad dressing.

3. Arrange salad on a bed of lettuce leaves. Garnish with tomato slices and parsley.

NUTRITION FACTS

Recipe yields 2 serving
Amount per serving
Calories 240
Total Fat 7 g
Total Carb 20 g
Protein 30 g
Sodium 188 mg

15. Lean Machine Trout Almandine

Ingredients

2 small trout
1/4 cup white wine
3/4 tsp butter
Juice of 1/2 lemon
1/8 cup slivered almonds
1 tbsp fresh parsley, chopped

Directions

1. Braise trout in white wine until done.

2. Remove trout, and drain off fat.

3. In the skillet, add butter and lemon juice, and saute almonds until lightly browned.

4. Mix in chopped parsley, and pour almond mixture over trout.

Serve immediately.

NUTRITION FACTS

Recipe yields 2 servings
Amount per serving
Calories 322
Total Fat 20 g
Total Car 5 g
Protein 26 g

Sodium 78 g

16. Buff Guy Chicken in White Wine Sauce

Ingredients

4 8-ounce chicken breasts
1/4 lbs fresh mushrooms, sliced
1/2 cup dry white wine
1 tsp lemon juice
1/2 tsp dried dill
1/2 cup evaporated skim milk
1/2 cup Italian bread crumbs

Directions

1. Place chicken breasts between two sheets of paper towels and pound flat.

2. Simmer mushrooms in white wine, lemon juice, and dill until white wine is almost evaporated.

3. Spread mushrooms on flattened chicken breasts, roll them up, and fasten them with toothpicks.

4. Roll breasts in evaporated milk and bread crumbs, completely covering chicken.

5. Arrange chicken in nonstick baking pan and bake in a 350 degree oven for 35 minutes or until chicken is tender.

NUTRITION FACTS

Recipe yields 4 serving
Amount per serving
Calories 251
Total Fat 6.6 g
Total Carb 29 g
Protein 25 g

17. Crazy Blueberry and Cottage Cheese

Ingredients

1 cup low-fat cottage cheese
1/4 cup skim milk
3/4 cup whole wheat flour
2 egg whites
1 1/2 teaspoons lemon juice
1 cup whole fresh blueberries

Directions

1. Combine cottage cheese, skim milk, and flour in a bowl.

2. Beat egg whites until frothy but not stiff and add to cottage cheese mixture.

3. Add lemon juice, stir, add blueberries, and stir again.

4. Pour all of the batter into a nonstick frying pan and turn when tops begin to bubble and bottom is lightly browned.

5. Divide into four wedges and serve.

NUTRITION FACTS

Recipe yields 4 servings
Amount per serving
Calories 154

Total Fat 1.4 g
Total Carb 24 g
Protein 11 g

18. Forearm Blasting Spinach Noodle Lasagna

Ingredients

1 pound spinach noodles
2 large onions, chopped
1 clove garlic, crushed
1/4 cup dry white wine or water
2 pounds lean ground beef
4 large ripe tomatoes, pureed
7 ounces salt-free tomato paste
2 tbsp each: chopped fresh parsley, basil, oregano
32 ounces Weight Watchers unsalted cottage cheese
2 egg whites
1 pound fresh spinach, chopped, cooked, and drained
1 large tomato, thinly sliced for garnish

Directions

1. Boil noodles until tender. Drain.

2. Braise onions and garlic in white wine for 4 minutes. Add ground beef. Cook until no longer pink. Drain fat.

3. Add pureed tomatoes, tomato paste, and herbs. Simmer for 20 minutes.

4. in a blender, mix cottage cheese, egg whites, and spinach. Puree.

5. Preheat oven to 350 degrees. Place a layer of meat sauce in a large baking pan. Layer with noodles and spinach mixture. Repeat layers, ending with noodles.

6. Arrange tomato slices on top. Bake for 45 minutes.

NUTRITION FACTS

Recipe yields 12 servings
Amount per serving
Calories 253
Total Fat 8 g
Total Carb 18 g
Protein 34 g
Sodium 84 mg

19. Eggs over Veggies

Ingredients

8 egg whites
3 tblsp minced onions
3/4 tsp garlic powder
3 tbsp water
Olive Oil
1 cup diced tomatoes
1 cup boiled and diced potatoes
1 cup diced zucchini

Directions

1. Beat egg whites, onion, garlic powder, and water until mixture is slightly frothy.

2. Coat bottom of a nonstick skillet with olive oil.

3. Cook and stir tomatoes, potatoes, and zucchini for 2 minutes in frying pan.

4. Pour egg mixture over vegetables.

5. As mixture begins to set at bottom and sides of the pan, gently lift cooked portions with spatula so that the uncooked portions can flow to the bottom of the pan.

6. Continue this process until eggs are thick and cooked but still moist.

NUTRITION FACTS

Recipe yields 2 servings
Amount per serving
Calories 67
Total Fat 1 g
Total Carb 8 g
Protein 3 g

20. Dude's Spinach Helper

Ingredients

1 1/2 tsp olive oil
1/2 onion, chopped
1/2 clove garlic, crushed
1/2 green onion, sliced
1/2 green pepper, chopped
1/2 pound lean ground beef
1/2 pound fresh mushrooms, sliced
5 ounces fresh spinach, washed and drained
1/2 cup nonfat yogurt
1 ounce dry curd, unsalted cottage cheese
1 ounce water
1 1/2 tsp fresh oregano

Directions

1. Heat olive oil in skillet. Saute onion, garlic, green onion, and green pepper until tender.

2. Add ground beef, and cook until just browned.

3. Add mushrooms and spinach. When spinach is limp, add remaining ingredients. Heat through and serve.

NUTRITION FACTS

Recipe yields 2 servings
Amount per serving
Calories 349
Total Fat 12 g

Total Carb 37 g
Protein 34 g
Sodium 151 mg

21. Chili Challenge

Ingredients

1 pound lean ground beef
1 onion, chopped
1 green pepper, chopped
3 tomatoes, chopped
1 teaspoon chili powder
1/2 teaspoon cumin powder
Dash ground red pepper
1 16-ounce can red kidney beans
1 15-ounce can chick-peas
1 15-ounce can corn, rinsed and drained
1 8-ounce can low-sodium tomato paste
6 ounces water

Directions

1. Cook ground beef in large skillet until no longer pink. Drain fat.

2. Add remaining ingredients, first rinsing and draining beans, chick-peas and corn.

3. Stir to ensure equal distribution.

4. Cover and simmer for 1 hour, stirring occasionally.

5. Keep leftover chili covered in the refrigerator. To reheat, add water to desired consistency, and stir occasionally until heated through.

NUTRITION FACTS

Recipe yields 8 servings
Amount per serving
Calories 329
Total Fat 8 g
Total Carb 44 g
Protein 23 g
Sodium 192 mg

22. Tricep Blasting Tuna Salad and Dill

Ingredients

1 7-ounce can of water-packed low-sodium tuna, rinsed and drained
1/4 cup chopped celery
1/4 cup chopped fresh dill
2 tbsp chopped fresh parsley
1/4 cup nonfat yogurt
1/2 tsp low-sodium Dijon mustard
Dash Pepper

Directions

1. Combine all ingredients in a mixing bowl.

2. Serve on lettuce, pita bread, baked potato, pasta or rice.

NUTRITION FACTS

Recipe yields 2 servings
Amount per serving
Calories 158
Total Fat 1 g
Total Carb 7 g
Protein 21 g
Sodium 158 mg

23. Lean Muscle Building Grilled Steak and Cheese

Ingredients

4 slices favorite bread
½ green pepper, sliced
½ small onion, sliced
2 slices reduced fat pepper jack cheese
8oz thinly sliced 5280meat sirloin tip steak
Steak seasoning of choice, optional

Directions

1. Season meat and cook as desired.

2. Add peppers and onions to medium skillet and cook until tender.

3. Layer steak, veggies and cheese onto bread.

4. Top with additional bread slice.

5. Heat medium skillet or grill pan over medium heat.

6. Add sandwich to pan and toast until golden.

7. Flip and toast until cheese is fully melted.

8. Serve

Nutrition Facts

Number of Servings: 2
Amount per serving
Calories 391
Protein 38.3g
Carbs 35.5g
Fat 9.5g
Fiber 7.3g

24. Insane Truffles

Ingredients

2 ½ scoops (100g) Strawberry Protein Powder
3/4 cup (80g) Oat Flour
2 tbsp. (14g) Coconut Flour
½ cup Reduced-Fat Shredded Coconut (can omit, if desired)
¼ cup Milk (+ 1-2 tbsp., if necessary)
2 tbsp. Honey
2 tbsp. Coconut Oil
½ tsp. Coconut Extract
¼ cup White Chocolate Chip

Directions.

1. Mix together protein, oat flour, coconut flour and shredded coconut.

2. Combine honey and coconut oil and heat in microwave until melted.

3. Mix milk into oil/honey.

4. Combine wet and dry ingredients (keep mixing – it will seem very dry at first, but put those arms to work and keep combining until a dough forms).

5. Cover your dough and chill for 30 minutes.

6. Roll dough into desired size truffles.

7. Roll truffles in melted white chocolate.

8. Allow to set in refrigerator or freezer until white chocolate is hard.

Nutrition Facts

Makes 20 Truffles
Number of Servings: 1
Amount Per Serving
Calories 87
Protein 4.2g
Carbs 8.2g
Fat 4.4g

25. Ripped Body Salmon Steaks and Quinoa

Ingredients

1 salmon steak (200g)
Asparagus & broccolini
1 cup cooked quinoa
2 tbs low fat Greek yoghurt
1 tsp capers
Squeeze of lemon

Directions

1. Cook quinoa for about 15 mins.

2. Cook salmon for 3 mins skin side up on a bbq grill plate or frying pan. Flip and cook for a further 1-2 mins (or to your liking).

3. Steam asparagus & broccolini.

4. Serve with capers, yoghurt and a squeeze of lemon.

Nutrition Facts

Servings 1

I don't know, but it has a lot of protein in it.

Conclusion

Here is a list of the items that I use in the recipes. Again you do not have to use them, any high quality alternative will work.

Amino IV

ISO Lean Pro 100% Premium Whey Protein Isolate

Protein Ice Cream Powder

Caramel Protein Bar

Quinoa

Thanks again for downloading this recipe book. I'm in the process of writing more recipe and other health and fitness books. Ever since I was a kid growing up in Texas, I have had a passion for working out and staying fit. I played Football in High School and then joined the United States Army where I became an Infantry Soldier. As an 11-Bravo part of my job was to be in and stay in top physical condition, 32 Years after joining the Army at the age of 18, my passion is still working out and staying fit and I plan to share what I know with you and others. So I am starting a free book club, which means whenever I launch a new book I will make it free for you to download via Amazon's Kindle Book Store. If you are interested in joining my free book club, let me know by sending me an email with "ad me to your free book club" in the subject. I will send you updates and information about upcoming books and products. readdragonpublishing@gmail.com

If you enjoyed this book, would you please leave a review for this book on Amazon? It'd be greatly appreciated!

Finally, if you find any problems or areas that you feel could be better in this book, please let me know so that I can address them. Again, you can reach me at readdragonpublishing@gmail.com

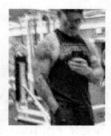

Thank you

Clark Moraign

www.ingramcontent.com/pod-product-compliance
Lightning Source LLC
LaVergne TN
LVHW051756250225

804528LV00002B/318